VEGAN RECIPES FOR RENAL HEALTH

Kidney-Friendly Plant-Based Meals to Help You Feel Your Best

Dr Lily Morgan

COPYRIGHT PAGE

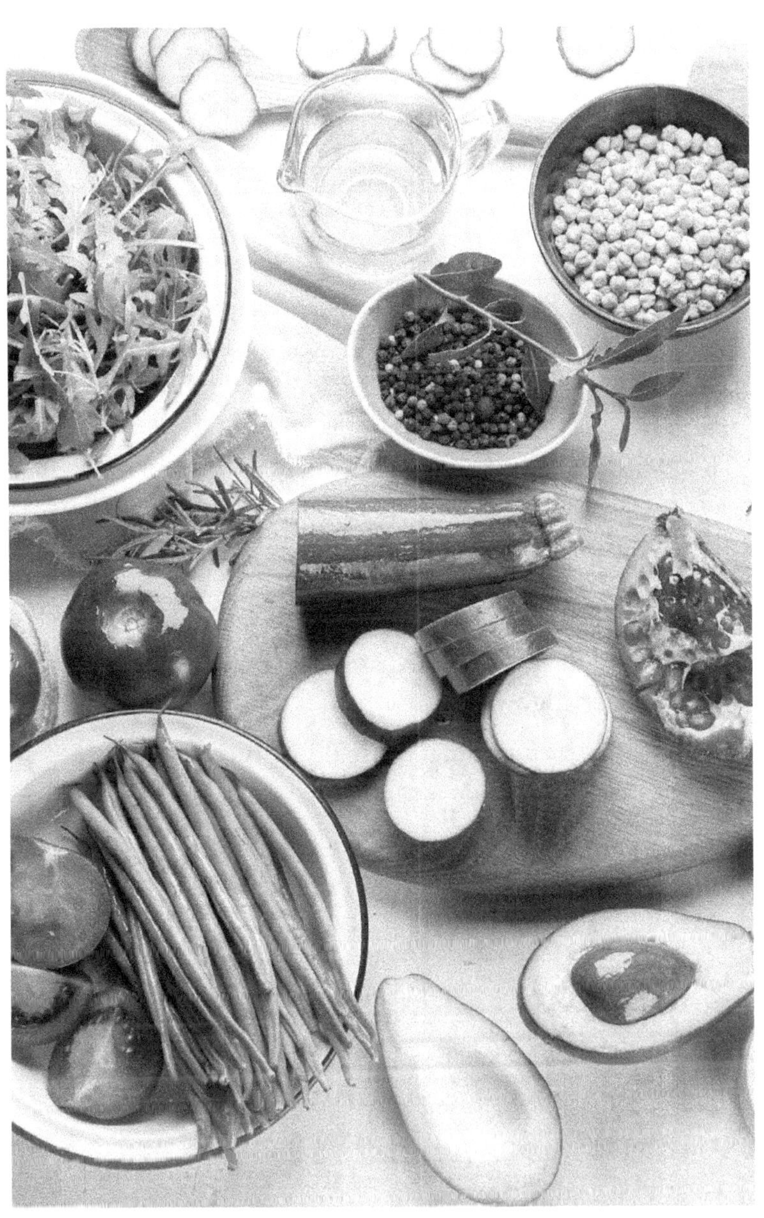

TABLE OF CONTENTS

Chapter 5: Snacks and Appetizers

Chapter 6: Desserts 97

INTRODUCTION

R enal health, often referred to as kidney health, is a critical aspect of overall well-being. The kidneys are remarkable organs responsible for a multitude of functions within the body, including filtering waste products from the blood, regulating blood pressure, and maintaining the body's fluid balance.

To truly appreciate the importance of renal health, it's essential to understand the intricate workings of these bean-shaped organs. The kidneys consist of tiny structures called nephrons, which serve as the filtration units. Each day, these nephrons filter around 120 to 150 quarts of blood to produce approximately 1 to 2 quarts of urine, eliminating waste and excess substances from the body. This natural detoxification process helps maintain internal equilibrium.

However, when renal health is compromised, this delicate balance can be disrupted. Kidney diseases and conditions can impair the kidneys' ability to function optimally. Factors such as high blood pressure, diabetes, and certain medications can contribute to kidney problems. Understanding the early signs of kidney issues, such as changes in urine output, persistent swelling, and unexplained fatigue, is crucial for early intervention.

One promising approach to supporting and even improving renal health is adopting a vegan diet. A vegan diet excludes all animal products, including meat, dairy, and eggs, and primarily relies on plant-based foods. This dietary choice offers several notable benefits for renal health:

1. Reduced Protein Load: Animal proteins, when broken down, produce waste products that the kidneys must filter. A vegan diet, lower in protein than the typical Western diet, eases the kidneys' workload, potentially slowing the progression of kidney disease.
2. Lower Blood Pressure: High blood pressure is a common risk factor for kidney damage. Vegan diets, rich in fruits, vegetables, and whole grains, have been shown to lower blood pressure, reducing the strain on the kidneys.

3. Decreased Inflammation: Chronic inflammation can harm kidney tissue. Plant-based diets are known for their anti-inflammatory properties, which can help protect renal health.

4. Improved Blood Sugar Control: For individuals with diabetes, a well-planned vegan diet can aid in better blood sugar control, reducing the risk of kidney complications associated with uncontrolled diabetes.

5. Enhanced Heart Health: A vegan diet often leads to improved cardiovascular health, reducing the risk of heart-related complications that can indirectly impact the kidneys.

In summary, understanding renal health and its intricate connection to diet is a vital step in maintaining overall well-being. A vegan diet, rich in plant-based foods and devoid of animal products, offers a promising path to supporting and potentially enhancing renal health. By embracing the benefits of a vegan lifestyle, individuals can take proactive steps towards safeguarding their kidneys and promoting longevity and vitality.

Chapter 1: 30-Day Meal Plan

Week 1:

Day 1:

- Breakfast: Vegan Berry Smoothie Bowl
- Lunch: Lentil and Vegetable Soup
- Dinner: Vegan Lentil Loaf
- Snacks: Guacamole with Veggie Sticks
- Dessert: Vegan Chocolate Avocado Mousse

Day 2:

- Breakfast: Avocado Toast with Tomato Salsa
- Lunch: Vegan Caesar Salad
- Dinner: Eggplant Parmesan
- Snacks: Vegan Spinach and Artichoke Dip
- Dessert: Vegan Banana Bread

Day 3:

- Breakfast: Quinoa Porridge with Almonds
- Lunch: Mediterranean Quinoa Salad
- Dinner: Vegan Thai Green Curry

- Snacks: Hummus with Pita Bread
- Dessert: Berry Crisp

Day 4:

- Breakfast: Sweet Potato and Spinach Breakfast Burrito
- Lunch: Chickpea and Spinach Curry
- Dinner: Mushroom Stroganoff
- Snacks: Vegan Salsa Verde
- Dessert: Vegan Chocolate Chip Cookies

Day 5:

- Breakfast: Blueberry Oat Pancakes
- Lunch: Vegan Wrap with Hummus
- Dinner: Vegan Ratatouille
- Snacks: Sweet Potato Fries
- Dessert: Vegan Rice Pudding

Day 6:

- Breakfast: Tofu Scramble with Vegetables
- Lunch: Spinach and Avocado Salad
- Dinner: Spicy Black Bean and Quinoa Bowl

- Snacks: Vegan Buffalo Cauliflower Bites
- Dessert: Vegan Blueberry Cheesecake

Day 7:

- Breakfast: Chia Seed Pudding with Mango
- Lunch: Vegan Rice Paper Rolls
- Dinner: Vegan Butternut Squash Risotto
- Snacks: Stuffed Mushrooms
- Dessert: Vegan Apple Crumble

Week 2:

Day 8:

- Breakfast: Vegan Breakfast Tacos
- Lunch: Quinoa and Black Bean Salad
- Dinner: Teriyaki Tofu Stir-Fry
- Snacks: Vegan Spring Rolls
- Dessert: Chocolate Covered Strawberries

Day 9:

- Breakfast: Overnight Oats with Berries
- Lunch: Vegan Minestrone Soup
- Dinner: Vegan Lasagna

- Snacks: Roasted Chickpeas
- Dessert: Vegan Pumpkin Pie

Day 10:

- Breakfast: Vegan French Toast
- Lunch: Tofu and Vegetable Stir-Fry
- Dinner: Cauliflower and Chickpea Curry
- Snacks: Vegan Caprese Skewers
- Dessert: Vegan Coconut Macaroons

Day 11:

- Breakfast: Green Smoothie with Kale and Banana
- Lunch: Vegan Nicoise Salad
- Dinner: Vegan Mushroom Risotto
- Snacks: Vegan Popcorn with Nutritional Yeast
- Dessert: Vegan Chocolate Fondue

Day 12:

- Breakfast: Coconut Yogurt Parfait
- Lunch: Sweet Potato and Chickpea Salad
- Dinner: Stuffed Bell Peppers
- Snacks: Spicy Vegan Nuts

- Dessert: Vegan Lemon Bars

Day 13:

- Breakfast: Vegan Breakfast Sandwich
- Lunch: Vegan Tofu Bahn Mi
- Dinner: Vegan Spaghetti Bolognese
- Snacks: Vegan Bruschetta
- Dessert: Vegan Peanut Butter Cups

Day 14:

- Breakfast: Peanut Butter Banana Oatmeal
- Lunch: Roasted Red Pepper and Lentil Soup
- Dinner: Vegan BBQ Jackfruit Sandwich
- Snacks: Vegan Cucumber Rolls
- Dessert: Vegan Strawberry Shortcake

Week 3:

Day 15:

- Breakfast: Veggie Breakfast Hash
- Lunch: Vegan Greek Salad
- Dinner: Vegan Lentil Loaf
- Snacks: Vegan Nachos

- Dessert: Vegan Carrot Cake

Day 16:

- Breakfast: Chickpea Flour Pancakes
- Lunch: Vegan Wrap with Hummus
- Dinner: Eggplant Parmesan
- Snacks: Vegan Potato Skins
- Dessert: Vegan Chocolate Pots de Crème

Day 17:

- Breakfast: Spinach and Mushroom Vegan Quiche
- Lunch: Spinach and Avocado Salad
- Dinner: Vegan Thai Green Curry
- Snacks: Vegan Tofu Satay
- Dessert: Vegan Black Bean Brownies

Day 18:

- Breakfast: Vegan Breakfast Burrito Bowl
- Lunch: Vegan Rice Paper Rolls
- Dinner: Mushroom Stroganoff
- Snacks: Guacamole with Veggie Sticks
- Dessert: Vegan Tiramisu

Day 19:

- Breakfast: Vegan Banana Bread
- Lunch: Quinoa and Black Bean Salad
- Dinner: Vegan Ratatouille
- Snacks: Vegan Spinach and Artichoke Dip
- Dessert: Berry Crisp

Day 20:

- Breakfast: Vegan Chocolate Avocado Mousse
- Lunch: Vegan Caesar Salad
- Dinner: Spicy Black Bean and Quinoa Bowl
- Snacks: Hummus with Pita Bread
- Dessert: Vegan Chocolate Chip Cookies

Day 21:

- Breakfast: Vegan Salsa Verde
- Lunch: Vegan Minestrone Soup
- Dinner: Vegan Lasagna
- Snacks: Sweet Potato Fries
- Dessert: Vegan Rice Pudding

Week 4:

Day 22:

- Breakfast: Vegan Blueberry Cheesecake
- Lunch: Tofu and Vegetable Stir-Fry
- Dinner: Cauliflower and Chickpea Curry
- Snacks: Vegan Caprese Skewers
- Dessert: Vegan Coconut Macaroons

Day 23:

- Breakfast: Chocolate Covered Strawberries
- Lunch: Vegan Nicoise Salad
- Dinner: Vegan Mushroom Risotto
- Snacks: Vegan Popcorn with Nutritional Yeast
- Dessert: Vegan Chocolate Fondue

Day 24:

- Breakfast: Vegan Apple Crumble
- Lunch: Sweet Potato and Chickpea Salad
- Dinner: Stuffed Bell Peppers
- Snacks: Spicy Vegan Nuts
- Dessert: Vegan Lemon Bars

Day 25:

- Breakfast: Vegan Chocolate Chip Cookies
- Lunch: Roasted Red Pepper and Lentil Soup
- Dinner: Vegan BBQ Jackfruit Sandwich
- Snacks: Vegan Cucumber Rolls
- Dessert: Vegan Strawberry Shortcake

Day 26:

- Breakfast: Vegan Peanut Butter Cups
- Lunch: Vegan Tofu Bahn Mi
- Dinner: Vegan Spaghetti Bolognese
- Snacks: Vegan Bruschetta
- Dessert: Vegan Carrot Cake

Day 27:

- Breakfast: Vegan Lemon Bars
- Lunch: Vegan Greek Salad
- Dinner: Vegan Lentil Loaf
- Snacks: Vegan Nachos
- Dessert: Vegan Chocolate Pots de Crème

Day 28:

- Breakfast: Vegan Black Bean Brownies
- Lunch: Vegan Wrap with Hummus
- Dinner: Eggplant Parmesan
- Snacks: Vegan Potato Skins
- Dessert: Vegan Tiramisu

Day 29:

- Breakfast: Vegan Tiramisu
- Lunch: Spinach and Avocado Salad
- Dinner: Vegan Thai Green Curry
- Snacks: Vegan Tofu Satay
- Dessert: Vegan Blueberry Cheesecake

Day 30:

- Breakfast: Vegan Carrot Cake
- Lunch: Quinoa and Black Bean Salad
- Dinner: Vegan Ratatouille
- Snacks: Vegan Spinach and Artichoke Dip
- Dessert: Berry Crisp

Congratulations on completing the 30-day vegan meal plan! This diverse selection of kidney-friendly recipes offers both nutrition and deliciousness while focusing on renal health. Feel free to adjust the plan to meet your specific dietary preferences and needs. Enjoy your meals!

Chapter 2: Breakfast Recipes

In this chapter, we're diving into a delightful array of vegan breakfast recipes that not only nourish your body but also tantalize your taste buds. These recipes are thoughtfully crafted to support renal health while delivering a burst of morning energy.

Vegan Berry Smoothie Bowl

Ingredients:

- 1 cup frozen mixed berries
- 1 ripe banana
- 1/2 cup almond milk
- 2 tbsp chia seeds
- 1/4 cup granola
- Fresh berries for topping

Instructions:

1. Blend frozen berries, banana, and almond milk until smooth.

2. Pour into a bowl and top with chia seeds, granola, and fresh berries.

3. Enjoy this vibrant, nutrient-packed start to your day!

Avocado Toast with Tomato Salsa

Ingredients:

- 2 slices whole-grain bread
- 1 ripe avocado
- 1 tomato, diced
- 1/4 red onion, finely chopped
- Fresh cilantro leaves
- Lime juice
- Salt and pepper to taste

Instructions:

1. Toast the bread to your preference.

2. Mash the avocado and spread it on the toasted bread.

3. In a bowl, mix diced tomato, red onion, cilantro, lime juice, salt, and pepper to create a zesty salsa.

4. Spoon the salsa over the avocado toast and savor the freshness.

Quinoa Porridge with Almonds

Ingredients:

- 1 cup quinoa
- 2 cups almond milk
- 1/4 cup sliced almonds
- 1 tbsp maple syrup
- Fresh berries for topping

Instructions:

1. Rinse quinoa under cold water and drain.
2. In a saucepan, combine quinoa and almond milk. Bring to a boil, then reduce heat and simmer for 15-20 minutes until quinoa is cooked and mixture thickens.
3. Stir in sliced almonds and maple syrup.
4. Serve with fresh berries on top for a wholesome breakfast.

Sweet Potato and Spinach Breakfast Burrito

Ingredients:

- 1 large sweet potato, diced
- 1 cup baby spinach
- 1/2 cup black beans, cooked
- 4 whole-grain tortillas
- Salsa of your choice

Instructions:

1. Roast the sweet potato cubes until tender.
2. In a pan, wilt the baby spinach.
3. Warm the tortillas.
4. Assemble burritos by placing sweet potatoes, spinach, and black beans in each tortilla.
5. Add salsa for extra flavor, roll them up, and enjoy!

Blueberry Oat Pancakes

Ingredients:

- 1 cup rolled oats
- 1 ripe banana

- 1/2 cup blueberries
- 1/2 cup almond milk
- 1 tsp baking powder
- 1 tsp vanilla extract

Instructions:

1. Blend oats, banana, blueberries, almond milk, baking powder, and vanilla extract until smooth.
2. Heat a non-stick pan over medium heat and ladle in the pancake batter.
3. Cook until bubbles form on the surface, then flip and cook until golden brown.
4. Serve with additional blueberries and a drizzle of maple syrup.

Tofu Scramble with Vegetables

Ingredients:

- 1/2 block of firm tofu, crumbled
- 1 cup mixed vegetables (bell peppers, onions, spinach)
- 1 tsp turmeric powder
- 1/2 tsp cumin

- Salt and pepper to taste

Instructions:

1. In a skillet, sauté mixed vegetables until tender.
2. Add crumbled tofu and spices, stir until tofu is heated through.
3. Season with salt and pepper.
4. A hearty, protein-packed scramble is ready to enjoy!

Chia Seed Pudding with Mango

Ingredients:

- 1/4 cup chia seeds
- 1 cup almond milk
- 1 ripe mango, diced
- 1 tbsp agave nectar or maple syrup
- Sliced almonds for garnish

Instructions:

1. Mix chia seeds and almond milk in a jar or bowl.
2. Stir in agave nectar or maple syrup and refrigerate for a few hours or overnight.

3. Top with diced mango and sliced almonds for a refreshing and nutritious pudding.

Vegan Breakfast Tacos

Ingredients:

- 4 small whole-grain tortillas
- 1 cup black beans, cooked
- 1 cup tofu, crumbled and seasoned with taco spices
- Sliced avocado
- Salsa
- Fresh cilantro

Instructions:

1. Warm the tortillas.
2. Fill each tortilla with black beans, seasoned tofu, sliced avocado, salsa, and a sprinkle of fresh cilantro.
3. Roll up and relish these protein-packed breakfast tacos.

Overnight Oats with Berries

Ingredients:

- 1 cup rolled oats
- 1 cup almond milk
- 1/2 cup mixed berries
- 1 tbsp honey or agave nectar
- Chopped nuts for topping

Instructions:

1. Combine oats and almond milk in a jar or bowl.
2. Add mixed berries and sweetener.
3. Refrigerate overnight.
4. In the morning, sprinkle chopped nuts on top for extra crunch and flavor.

Vegan French Toast

Ingredients:

- 4 slices of whole-grain bread
- 1 ripe banana
- 1/2 cup almond milk
- 1 tsp cinnamon

- 1 tsp vanilla extract

Instructions:

1. Mash the banana and mix it with almond milk, cinnamon, and vanilla extract.
2. Dip each slice of bread into the mixture and cook in a non-stick pan until golden brown.
3. Serve with fresh fruit or a drizzle of maple syrup.

Green Smoothie with Kale and Banana

Ingredients:

- 1 cup kale leaves, stems removed
- 1 ripe banana
- 1/2 cup pineapple chunks
- 1/2 cup almond milk
- 1 tbsp chia seeds

Instructions:

1. Blend kale, banana, pineapple, and almond milk until smooth.

2. Sprinkle chia seeds on top for added fiber and omega-3s.

3. Start your day with a vibrant green smoothie to boost your energy and nutrition.

Coconut Yogurt Parfait

Ingredients:

- 1 cup coconut yogurt
- 1/2 cup granola
- 1/2 cup mixed berries
- Drizzle of agave nectar or honey

Instructions:

1. In a glass or bowl, layer coconut yogurt, granola, mixed berries, and drizzle with agave nectar or honey.

2. Repeat for a delicious and visually appealing parfait.

Vegan Breakfast Sandwich

Ingredients:

- 2 whole-grain English muffins

- Vegan sausage patties

- Sliced tomato

- Lettuce leaves

- Vegan cheese (optional)

- Vegan mayo or avocado spread

Instructions:

1. Cook vegan sausage patties according to package instructions.

2. Assemble sandwiches with sausage, tomato, lettuce, cheese (if desired), and spread of choice.

3. Enjoy a hearty and savory breakfast on the go.

Peanut Butter Banana Oatmeal

Ingredients:

- 1 cup rolled oats

- 2 cups almond milk

- 2 ripe bananas, sliced

- 2 tbsp peanut butter

- 1 tbsp maple syrup

Instructions:

1. Combine oats and almond milk in a pot, bring to a simmer, and cook until oats are tender.

2. Stir in sliced bananas, peanut butter, and maple syrup.

3. Dive into this creamy and satisfying oatmeal.

Veggie Breakfast Hash

Ingredients:

- 2 cups diced potatoes
- 1 cup bell peppers, diced
- 1 cup zucchini, diced
- 1/2 cup red onion, chopped
- 1 tsp paprika
- Salt and pepper to taste

Instructions:

1. In a skillet, sauté potatoes, bell peppers, zucchini, and red onion until golden and tender.

2. Season with paprika, salt, and pepper.

3. This flavorful veggie hash is a great way to start your day with a dose of veggies.

Chapter 3: Lunch Recipes

For a satisfying and nutritious midday meal, explore this collection of delightful lunch recipes that are not only good for your renal health but also bursting with flavor. These recipes encompass a variety of vegan options, from hearty soups to refreshing salads and savory stir-fries.

Lentil and Vegetable Soup

Ingredients:

- 1 cup dried green lentils
- 4 cups vegetable broth
- 1 onion, diced
- 2 carrots, chopped
- 2 celery stalks, chopped
- 1 red bell pepper, diced
- 1 zucchini, diced
- 2 cloves garlic, minced
- 1 teaspoon dried thyme
- 1 teaspoon dried rosemary
- Salt and pepper to taste

- Fresh parsley for garnish

Instructions:

1. In a large pot, sauté the onions, carrots, and celery until they begin to soften.
2. Add the garlic, thyme, and rosemary, and cook for another minute.
3. Stir in the lentils, vegetable broth, and the remaining vegetables.
4. Bring the soup to a boil, then reduce the heat and simmer for about 30 minutes or until the lentils and vegetables are tender.
5. Season with salt and pepper, and garnish with fresh parsley before serving.

Vegan Caesar Salad

Ingredients:

- 1 head of romaine lettuce, chopped
- 1 cup croutons (ensure they're vegan)
- 1/4 cup vegan Caesar dressing
- 1/4 cup vegan Parmesan cheese
- 1 lemon, juiced

- 2 tablespoons olive oil

- 1 clove garlic, minced

- Salt and pepper to taste

Instructions:

1. In a small bowl, whisk together the lemon juice, olive oil, minced garlic, salt, and pepper to make the dressing.

2. In a large salad bowl, combine the chopped romaine lettuce and croutons.

3. Drizzle the Caesar dressing over the salad and toss to coat.

4. Sprinkle vegan Parmesan cheese on top before serving.

Mediterranean Quinoa Salad

Ingredients:

- 1 cup quinoa, rinsed and cooked

- 1 cup cherry tomatoes, halved

- 1 cucumber, diced

- 1/2 red onion, finely chopped

- 1/2 cup Kalamata olives, pitted and sliced

- 1/2 cup fresh parsley, chopped

- 1/4 cup extra-virgin olive oil

- 2 tablespoons red wine vinegar

- Salt and pepper to taste

Instructions:

1. In a large bowl, combine the cooked quinoa, cherry tomatoes, cucumber, red onion, olives, and parsley.

2. In a separate small bowl, whisk together the olive oil, red wine vinegar, salt, and pepper to create the dressing.

3. Drizzle the dressing over the salad and toss to combine.

4. Serve chilled.

Chickpea and Spinach Curry

Ingredients:

- 1 can (15 oz) chickpeas, drained and rinsed

- 1 onion, finely chopped

- 2 cloves garlic, minced

- 1-inch piece of ginger, grated

- 1 can (14 oz) diced tomatoes

- 2 cups fresh spinach leaves
- 2 teaspoons curry powder
- 1 teaspoon ground cumin
- 1 teaspoon ground coriander
- 1/2 teaspoon turmeric
- 1/4 teaspoon cayenne pepper (adjust to taste)
- Salt and pepper to taste
- 1 tablespoon vegetable oil
- Fresh cilantro for garnish

Instructions:

1. In a large skillet, heat the vegetable oil over medium heat. Add the chopped onion and sauté until translucent.
2. Stir in the minced garlic, grated ginger, and spices (curry powder, cumin, coriander, turmeric, cayenne pepper). Cook for 1-2 minutes until fragrant.
3. Add the diced tomatoes (with their juices) and chickpeas to the skillet. Simmer for about 10 minutes, allowing the flavors to meld.
4. Stir in the fresh spinach and cook until wilted.
5. Season with salt and pepper to taste.

6. Serve the chickpea and spinach curry over rice or with naan bread, garnished with fresh cilantro.

Vegan Wrap with Hummus

Ingredients:

- 4 large whole-grain tortillas
- 1 cup hummus
- 1 cup shredded carrots
- 1 cup cucumber, thinly sliced
- 1 cup bell peppers (any color), thinly sliced
- 1 cup baby spinach leaves
- Salt and pepper to taste

Instructions:

1. Lay out the tortillas on a clean surface.
2. Spread a generous amount of hummus evenly over each tortilla.
3. Layer the shredded carrots, cucumber, bell peppers, and baby spinach on top of the hummus.
4. Season with salt and pepper to taste.
5. Roll up the tortillas tightly, tucking in the sides as you go.

6. Slice each wrap in half diagonally before serving.

Spinach and Avocado Salad

Ingredients:

- 6 cups fresh spinach leaves
- 1 avocado, sliced
- 1/2 cup cherry tomatoes, halved
- 1/4 cup red onion, thinly sliced
- 1/4 cup sliced almonds
- 2 tablespoons balsamic vinegar
- 2 tablespoons olive oil
- Salt and pepper to taste

Instructions:

1. In a large salad bowl, combine the fresh spinach leaves, sliced avocado, cherry tomatoes, red onion, and sliced almonds.
2. In a small bowl, whisk together the balsamic vinegar and olive oil to create the dressing.
3. Drizzle the dressing over the salad and toss gently to coat.
4. Season with salt and pepper to taste.

Vegan Rice Paper Rolls

Ingredients:

- 8 rice paper wrappers
- 1 cup cooked rice noodles
- 1 cup thinly sliced red bell pepper
- 1 cup thinly sliced cucumber
- 1 cup fresh cilantro leaves
- 1 cup fresh mint leaves
- 1 cup firm tofu, sliced into thin strips
- Peanut dipping sauce (store-bought or homemade)

Instructions:

1. Fill a large shallow bowl with warm water. Dip one rice paper wrapper into the water for about 5-10 seconds until it softens and becomes pliable.
2. Lay the softened rice paper on a clean, damp kitchen towel.
3. Layer a small amount of cooked rice noodles, red bell pepper, cucumber, cilantro, mint, and tofu on the lower third of the rice paper.
4. Fold the sides of the rice paper over the filling, then roll it up tightly from the bottom to form a spring roll.

5. Repeat the process with the remaining rice paper wrappers and ingredients.

6. Serve the rice paper rolls with peanut dipping sauce for a refreshing and healthy lunch option.

Spaghetti Aglio e Olio

Ingredients:

- 8 oz whole wheat spaghetti (or gluten-free spaghetti if preferred)
- 4 cloves garlic, thinly sliced
- 1/4 cup olive oil
- 1/4 teaspoon red pepper flakes (adjust to taste)
- 1/4 cup fresh parsley, chopped
- Salt and black pepper to taste
- Vegan Parmesan cheese (optional)

Instructions:

1. Cook the spaghetti according to package instructions until al dente. Drain and set aside.

2. In a large skillet, heat the olive oil over low-medium heat. Add the sliced garlic and red pepper flakes.

Sauté until the garlic is lightly golden (be careful not to burn it).

3. Toss the cooked spaghetti into the skillet with the garlic and olive oil. Stir to coat the pasta evenly.
4. Season with salt and black pepper to taste.
5. Remove from heat and sprinkle fresh parsley over the pasta.
6. If desired, serve with a sprinkle of vegan Parmesan cheese.

Quinoa and Black Bean Salad

Ingredients:

- 1 cup quinoa, rinsed and cooked
- 1 can (15 oz) black beans, drained and rinsed
- 1 cup corn kernels (fresh or frozen)
- 1 red bell pepper, diced
- 1/4 cup red onion, finely chopped
- 1/4 cup fresh cilantro, chopped
- Juice of 2 limes
- 2 tablespoons olive oil
- 1 teaspoon ground cumin
- Salt and pepper to taste

- Avocado slices for garnish (optional)

Instructions:

1. In a large bowl, combine the cooked quinoa, black beans, corn, red bell pepper, red onion, and fresh cilantro.

2. In a small bowl, whisk together the lime juice, olive oil, ground cumin, salt, and pepper to make the dressing.

3. Drizzle the dressing over the salad and toss to coat.

4. Garnish with avocado slices if desired.

Vegan Minestrone Soup

Ingredients:

- 1 tablespoon olive oil
- 1 onion, chopped
- 2 cloves garlic, minced
- 2 carrots, diced
- 2 celery stalks, diced
- 1 zucchini, diced
- 1 can (15 oz) diced tomatoes
- 1 can (15 oz) cannellini beans, drained and rinsed

- 6 cups vegetable broth

- 1 cup whole wheat pasta (small shapes)

- 2 teaspoons dried Italian seasoning

- Salt and black pepper to taste

- Fresh basil leaves for garnish (optional)

Instructions:

1. In a large pot, heat the olive oil over medium heat. Add the chopped onion and sauté until translucent.

2. Stir in the minced garlic, carrots, celery, and zucchini. Cook for a few minutes until the vegetables begin to soften.

3. Add the diced tomatoes, cannellini beans, vegetable broth, dried Italian seasoning, salt, and black pepper.

4. Bring the soup to a boil, then reduce the heat and simmer for about 15 minutes.

5. Stir in the whole wheat pasta and continue to simmer until the pasta is cooked.

6. Serve hot, garnished with fresh basil leaves if desired.

Tofu and Vegetable Stir-Fry

Ingredients:

- 1 block of extra-firm tofu, cubed
- 2 tablespoons soy sauce (or tamari for gluten-free)
- 1 tablespoon rice vinegar
- 1 tablespoon maple syrup
- 2 tablespoons vegetable oil
- 1 red bell pepper, sliced
- 1 yellow bell pepper, sliced
- 1 cup broccoli florets
- 1 cup snap peas
- 1 carrot, sliced into thin strips
- 2 cloves garlic, minced
- 1 tablespoon fresh ginger, minced
- Cooked brown rice for serving

Instructions:

1. In a small bowl, mix together the soy sauce, rice vinegar, and maple syrup to make the sauce.
2. Heat 1 tablespoon of vegetable oil in a large skillet over medium-high heat. Add the cubed tofu and cook

until golden brown on all sides. Remove from the skillet and set aside.

3. In the same skillet, add the remaining tablespoon of vegetable oil. Stir in the minced garlic and ginger and cook for about 30 seconds until fragrant.

4. Add the sliced bell peppers, broccoli, snap peas, and carrot strips to the skillet. Stir-fry for 5-7 minutes until the vegetables are tender-crisp.

5. Return the cooked tofu to the skillet and pour the sauce over the tofu and vegetables. Stir-fry for another 2-3 minutes to heat everything through.

6. Serve the tofu and vegetable stir-fry over cooked brown rice.

Vegan Nicoise Salad

Ingredients:

- 4 cups mixed greens
- 1 cup cherry tomatoes, halved
- 1 cup cooked green beans, cooled
- 1 cup cooked and quartered baby potatoes, cooled
- 1/2 cup Kalamata olives, pitted
- 1/4 cup red onion, thinly sliced

- 1 cup canned chickpeas, drained and rinsed

- 1/4 cup capers

- Lemon-tahini dressing (combine lemon juice, tahini, olive oil, and a pinch of salt)

Instructions:

1. Arrange the mixed greens on a large serving platter.

2. Arrange the cherry tomatoes, green beans, baby potatoes, Kalamata olives, red onion, chickpeas, and capers on top of the greens in an aesthetically pleasing manner.

3. Drizzle the lemon-tahini dressing over the salad before serving.

Sweet Potato and Chickpea Salad

Ingredients:

- 2 large sweet potatoes, peeled and diced

- 1 can (15 oz) chickpeas, drained and rinsed

- 2 tablespoons olive oil

- 1 teaspoon smoked paprika

- 1/2 teaspoon cumin

- Salt and black pepper to taste

- 4 cups fresh arugula
- 1/4 cup dried cranberries
- 1/4 cup chopped pecans
- Balsamic vinaigrette dressing

Instructions:

1. Preheat your oven to 400°F (200°C).
2. Toss the diced sweet potatoes and chickpeas with olive oil, smoked paprika, cumin, salt, and black pepper. Spread them out on a baking sheet and roast for about 25-30 minutes or until sweet potatoes are tender and slightly crispy.
3. Let the roasted sweet potatoes and chickpeas cool slightly.
4. Arrange the fresh arugula on a serving platter. Top with the roasted sweet potatoes, chickpeas, dried cranberries, and chopped pecans.
5. Drizzle with balsamic vinaigrette dressing before serving.

Vegan Tofu Bahn Mi

Ingredients:

- 1 baguette or 4 small baguette rolls
- 1 block of extra-firm tofu, sliced into thin strips
- 2 tablespoons soy sauce
- 1 tablespoon maple syrup
- 1 tablespoon rice vinegar
- 2 tablespoons vegetable oil
- 1/2 cup vegan mayonnaise
- 2 tablespoons sriracha sauce (adjust to taste)
- Pickled daikon radish and carrot (store-bought or homemade)
- Fresh cilantro sprigs
- Thinly sliced cucumber
- Sliced jalapeños (optional)

Instructions:

1. In a small bowl, mix together the soy sauce, maple syrup, rice vinegar, and vegetable oil to create a marinade for the tofu.

2. Marinate the tofu slices in this mixture for about 15 minutes.

3. Heat a skillet over medium-high heat and add the marinated tofu. Cook until it's browned and crispy on both sides.

4. In a separate small bowl, combine the vegan mayonnaise and sriracha sauce to make the spicy mayo.

5. Slice the baguette(s) in half lengthwise and spread the spicy mayo on both sides.

6. Layer the cooked tofu, pickled daikon radish and carrot, fresh cilantro sprigs, sliced cucumber, and jalapeños (if desired) inside the baguette(s).

7. Serve the vegan tofu Bahn Mi sandwiches immediately.

Roasted Red Pepper and Lentil Soup

Ingredients:

- 2 red bell peppers, roasted, peeled, and chopped
- 1 cup dried red lentils, rinsed and drained
- 1 onion, chopped
- 2 cloves garlic, minced
- 1 teaspoon ground cumin
- 1/2 teaspoon smoked paprika

- 6 cups vegetable broth
- Salt and black pepper to taste
- Fresh parsley for garnish

Instructions:

1. In a large pot, sauté the chopped onion until translucent.
2. Add the minced garlic, ground cumin, and smoked paprika. Cook for about a minute until fragrant.
3. Add the roasted red peppers, red lentils, and vegetable broth to the pot. Bring to a boil.
4. Reduce heat and simmer for about 20-25 minutes, or until the lentils are soft.
5. Use an immersion blender to puree the soup until smooth. Alternatively, carefully transfer the soup in batches to a blender to blend until smooth.
6. Season with salt and black pepper to taste.
7. Serve the roasted red pepper and lentil soup garnished with fresh parsley.

Vegan Sushi Bowl

Ingredients:

- 2 cups cooked sushi rice
- 1 cup cucumber, diced
- 1/2 cup carrots, julienned
- 1/2 cup avocado, sliced
- 1/4 cup pickled ginger
- 1/4 cup nori seaweed, chopped into strips
- 1/4 cup soy sauce (or tamari for gluten-free)
- 1 tablespoon sesame seeds
- Wasabi and soy sauce for serving

Instructions:

1. Divide the cooked sushi rice among serving bowls.
2. Arrange cucumber, carrots, avocado, pickled ginger, and nori seaweed on top of the rice in each bowl.
3. Drizzle soy sauce over the bowl and sprinkle with sesame seeds.
4. Serve with wasabi and extra soy sauce on the side.

Vegan Chili

Ingredients:

- 1 tablespoon olive oil
- 1 onion, chopped
- 2 cloves garlic, minced
- 1 bell pepper, diced
- 1 carrot, diced
- 1 zucchini, diced
- 1 can (15 oz) diced tomatoes
- 1 can (15 oz) kidney beans, drained and rinsed
- 1 can (15 oz) black beans, drained and rinsed
- 2 cups vegetable broth
- 2 tablespoons chili powder
- 1 teaspoon ground cumin
- 1 teaspoon paprika
- Salt and black pepper to taste
- Fresh cilantro for garnish (optional)

Instructions:

1. In a large pot, heat the olive oil over medium heat. Add the chopped onion and sauté until translucent.

2. Stir in the minced garlic, diced bell pepper, carrot, and zucchini. Cook for a few minutes until the vegetables start to soften.

3. Add the diced tomatoes, kidney beans, black beans, vegetable broth, chili powder, ground cumin, paprika, salt, and black pepper.

4. Bring the chili to a boil, then reduce the heat and let it simmer for about 20-30 minutes, stirring occasionally.

5. Taste and adjust seasoning if needed.

6. Serve the vegan chili hot, garnished with fresh cilantro if desired.

Vegan Greek Salad

Ingredients:

- 4 cups chopped romaine lettuce
- 1 cucumber, diced
- 1 cup cherry tomatoes, halved
- 1/2 cup red onion, thinly sliced
- 1/4 cup Kalamata olives, pitted and sliced
- 1/4 cup fresh parsley, chopped

- 1/4 cup vegan feta cheese, crumbled (store-bought or homemade)
- Greek salad dressing (combine olive oil, red wine vinegar, lemon juice, dried oregano, and salt to taste)

Instructions:

1. In a large salad bowl, combine the chopped romaine lettuce, diced cucumber, cherry tomatoes, red onion, Kalamata olives, and fresh parsley.
2. Sprinkle the vegan feta cheese over the salad.
3. Drizzle the Greek salad dressing over the salad and toss gently to coat.
4. Serve this refreshing Vegan Greek Salad immediately.

Chapter 4: Dinner Recipes

In this chapter, you'll discover a delightful array of vegan dinner recipes designed to tantalize your taste buds while keeping your renal health in mind. These recipes are carefully crafted to provide a balance of flavors and nutrients. Let's dive into these savory dishes:

Vegan Lentil Loaf

Ingredients:

- 1 cup green lentils, cooked and drained
- 1/2 cup rolled oats
- 1/2 cup finely chopped onions
- 1/2 cup finely chopped carrots
- 1/2 cup finely chopped celery
- 2 cloves garlic, minced
- 1/4 cup tomato sauce
- 1 tsp thyme
- 1 tsp rosemary
- Salt and pepper to taste

Instructions:

1. Preheat your oven to 350°F (175°C).

2. In a pan, sauté onions, carrots, celery, and garlic until tender.

3. In a mixing bowl, combine cooked lentils, oats, sautéed vegetables, tomato sauce, thyme, rosemary, salt, and pepper.

4. Press the mixture into a loaf pan and bake for 30-40 minutes until it's firm and slightly crispy on top.

Eggplant Parmesan

Ingredients:

- 2 large eggplants, sliced into rounds
- 1 cup vegan breadcrumbs
- 1/2 cup vegan parmesan cheese
- 2 cups marinara sauce
- 2 cups vegan mozzarella cheese
- Fresh basil leaves for garnish
- Olive oil for frying

Instructions:

1. Dip eggplant slices in olive oil and coat with breadcrumbs and vegan parmesan cheese.
2. In a pan, fry the coated eggplant slices until golden brown.
3. Preheat your oven to 375°F (190°C).
4. In a baking dish, layer marinara sauce, fried eggplant, and vegan mozzarella cheese.
5. Repeat the layers and finish with a layer of cheese on top.
6. Bake for 25-30 minutes or until bubbly and golden.
7. Garnish with fresh basil leaves before serving.

Vegan Thai Green Curry

Ingredients:

- 1 cup sliced mixed vegetables (e.g., bell peppers, zucchini, carrots)
- 1 can (14 oz) coconut milk
- 2 tbsp green curry paste
- 1 tbsp soy sauce
- 1 tbsp brown sugar
- 1 cup tofu cubes

- Fresh basil leaves for garnish
- Cooked jasmine rice

Instructions:

1. In a pan, heat coconut milk and green curry paste, stirring until fragrant.
2. Add sliced vegetables, soy sauce, and brown sugar. Simmer until veggies are tender.
3. Add tofu cubes and cook until heated through.
4. Serve over jasmine rice, garnished with fresh basil leaves.

Mushroom Stroganoff

Ingredients:

- 8 oz (225g) mushrooms, sliced
- 1 onion, finely chopped
- 2 cloves garlic, minced
- 1 cup vegetable broth
- 2 tbsp all-purpose flour
- 1 cup vegan sour cream
- 1 tsp paprika
- Salt and pepper to taste

- Cooked egg-free noodles or rice

Instructions:

1. In a large skillet, sauté the mushrooms, onions, and garlic until the mushrooms release their moisture and start to brown.
2. Sprinkle flour over the mushroom mixture and stir for a minute.
3. Pour in the vegetable broth and stir until the mixture thickens.
4. Reduce heat, add vegan sour cream, paprika, salt, and pepper. Stir until heated through.
5. Serve the mushroom stroganoff over cooked noodles or rice.

Vegan Ratatouille

Ingredients:

- 1 large eggplant, sliced
- 2 zucchinis, sliced
- 2 bell peppers, sliced
- 4 tomatoes, sliced
- 1 onion, thinly sliced

- 3 cloves garlic, minced

- 2 tsp dried thyme

- 2 tsp dried rosemary

- Salt and pepper to taste

- Olive oil

Instructions:

1. Preheat your oven to 375°F (190°C).

2. In a baking dish, arrange the sliced vegetables in an overlapping pattern.

3. Sprinkle garlic, thyme, rosemary, salt, and pepper over the vegetables.

4. Drizzle with olive oil and cover with foil.

5. Bake for 45-55 minutes or until the vegetables are tender.

Spicy Black Bean and Quinoa Bowl

Ingredients:

- 1 cup cooked quinoa

- 1 can (15 oz) black beans, drained and rinsed

- 1 cup corn kernels

- 1 cup cherry tomatoes, halved

- 1 avocado, diced

- 1/4 cup chopped cilantro

- 1 lime, juiced

- 1 tsp chili powder

- Salt and pepper to taste

Instructions:

1. In a large bowl, combine quinoa, black beans, corn, cherry tomatoes, and avocado.

2. In a small bowl, mix lime juice, chili powder, salt, and pepper.

3. Drizzle the lime dressing over the bowl.

4. Garnish with chopped cilantro before serving.

Vegan Butternut Squash Risotto

Ingredients:

- 2 cups arborio rice

- 4 cups vegetable broth

- 1 small butternut squash, diced

- 1 onion, finely chopped

- 2 cloves garlic, minced

- 1/2 cup dry white wine

- 1/2 cup nutritional yeast (for a cheesy flavor)
- 2 tbsp olive oil
- Salt and pepper to taste

Instructions:

1. In a large pot, heat the olive oil over medium heat. Add the onion and garlic, sauté until translucent.
2. Add the diced butternut squash and arborio rice. Stir for a few minutes.
3. Pour in the white wine and let it simmer until absorbed.
4. Gradually add the vegetable broth, one cup at a time, stirring frequently until absorbed.
5. Continue this process until the rice is creamy and cooked, about 20-25 minutes.
6. Stir in nutritional yeast, salt, and pepper.
7. Serve hot.

Teriyaki Tofu Stir-Fry

Ingredients:

- 1 block extra firm tofu, cubed
- 2 cups broccoli florets

- 1 red bell pepper, sliced

- 1/2 cup sliced carrots

- 1/4 cup teriyaki sauce (ensure it's vegan)

- 2 tbsp sesame oil

- 2 cloves garlic, minced

- Cooked brown rice

Instructions:

1. In a large skillet, heat the sesame oil over medium-high heat.

2. Add the tofu cubes and cook until golden on all sides.

3. Remove tofu from the skillet and set aside.

4. In the same skillet, sauté garlic and vegetables until tender.

5. Return the tofu to the skillet, pour teriyaki sauce over the mixture, and stir well.

6. Serve over cooked brown rice.

Vegan Lasagna

Ingredients:

- 9 lasagna noodles, cooked

- 2 cups marinara sauce

- 1 cup vegan ricotta cheese
- 1 cup spinach, chopped
- 1 cup vegan mozzarella cheese
- 1/4 cup vegan parmesan cheese
- 1 tsp dried oregano
- Salt and pepper to taste

Instructions:

1. Preheat your oven to 375°F (190°C).
2. In a baking dish, spread a thin layer of marinara sauce.
3. Place three cooked lasagna noodles on top.
4. Spread half of the vegan ricotta cheese, followed by half of the chopped spinach.
5. Sprinkle with vegan mozzarella, vegan parmesan, dried oregano, salt, and pepper.
6. Repeat the layers with remaining ingredients.
7. Finish with a final layer of noodles, marinara sauce, and a generous sprinkle of vegan mozzarella and parmesan cheese.
8. Bake for 25-30 minutes or until bubbly and golden.

Cauliflower and Chickpea Curry

Ingredients:

- 1 cauliflower, cut into florets
- 1 can (15 oz) chickpeas, drained and rinsed
- 1 onion, finely chopped
- 2 cloves garlic, minced
- 1 can (14 oz) coconut milk
- 2 tbsp curry powder
- 1 tsp turmeric
- Salt and pepper to taste
- Fresh cilantro for garnish
- Cooked basmati rice

Instructions:

1. In a large pot, sauté the onion and garlic until softened.
2. Add curry powder and turmeric, stirring for a minute.
3. Add cauliflower florets, chickpeas, and coconut milk.
4. Simmer until the cauliflower is tender and the sauce has thickened.
5. Season with salt and pepper.

6. Serve over basmati rice, garnished with fresh cilantro.

Vegan Mushroom Risotto

Ingredients:

- 1 1/2 cups Arborio rice
- 1 cup sliced mushrooms (variety of your choice)
- 1 onion, finely chopped
- 2 cloves garlic, minced
- 4 cups vegetable broth
- 1/2 cup dry white wine
- 1/4 cup nutritional yeast
- 2 tbsp olive oil
- Salt and pepper to taste
- Fresh parsley for garnish

Instructions:

1. In a large pot, heat the olive oil over medium heat. Add the onion and garlic, sauté until translucent.
2. Add the sliced mushrooms and cook until they release their moisture and turn golden brown.

3. Stir in the Arborio rice and cook for a couple of minutes.

4. Pour in the white wine and stir until it's mostly absorbed.

5. Gradually add the vegetable broth, one cup at a time, stirring frequently until the rice is creamy and cooked, about 20-25 minutes.

6. Stir in nutritional yeast, salt, and pepper.

7. Garnish with fresh parsley before serving.

Stuffed Bell Peppers

Ingredients:

- 4 large bell peppers, any color
- 1 cup cooked quinoa
- 1 can (15 oz) black beans, drained and rinsed
- 1 cup corn kernels
- 1 cup diced tomatoes
- 1/2 cup vegan shredded cheese
- 1 tsp cumin
- Salt and pepper to taste
- Fresh cilantro for garnish

Instructions:

1. Preheat your oven to 375°F (190°C).
2. Cut the tops off the bell peppers and remove the seeds and membranes.
3. In a large bowl, mix cooked quinoa, black beans, corn, diced tomatoes, vegan shredded cheese, cumin, salt, and pepper.
4. Stuff the mixture into the bell peppers.
5. Place the stuffed peppers in a baking dish, cover with foil, and bake for 30-40 minutes or until the peppers are tender.
6. Garnish with fresh cilantro before serving.

Vegan Spaghetti Bolognese

Ingredients:

- 8 oz (225g) spaghetti
- 1 cup lentils, cooked and drained
- 1 can (14 oz) crushed tomatoes
- 1 onion, finely chopped
- 2 cloves garlic, minced
- 1 carrot, grated
- 1 celery stalk, finely chopped

- 1 tsp dried basil

- 1 tsp dried oregano

- Salt and pepper to taste

- Fresh basil leaves for garnish

Instructions:

1. Cook the spaghetti according to package instructions until al dente. Drain and set aside.

2. In a large pan, sauté the onion, garlic, carrot, and celery until softened.

3. Add cooked lentils, crushed tomatoes, dried basil, dried oregano, salt, and pepper. Simmer for about 15 minutes.

4. Serve the lentil Bolognese sauce over the cooked spaghetti.

5. Garnish with fresh basil leaves.

Vegan BBQ Jackfruit Sandwich

Ingredients:

- 1 can (20 oz) young green jackfruit in brine, drained and shredded

- 1 cup BBQ sauce (ensure it's vegan)

- 4 whole wheat hamburger buns

- Coleslaw (vegan) for topping (optional)

- Pickles for garnish (optional)

Instructions:

1. In a pan, heat the shredded jackfruit and BBQ sauce over medium heat until heated through.

2. Toast the whole wheat buns.

3. Assemble the sandwiches by placing a generous portion of BBQ jackfruit on the bun.

4. Top with coleslaw and pickles if desired.

5. Serve with a side of your choice, like sweet potato fries or a salad.

Vegan Sweet Potato and Black Bean Enchiladas

Ingredients:

- 2 large sweet potatoes, peeled and diced

- 1 can (15 oz) black beans, drained and rinsed

- 1 cup corn kernels

- 1 cup diced tomatoes

- 1 tsp chili powder

- 1 tsp cumin

- Salt and pepper to taste

- 8 whole wheat tortillas

- 1 cup vegan enchilada sauce

- 1 cup vegan shredded cheese

- Fresh cilantro for garnish

Instructions:

1. Preheat your oven to 375°F (190°C).

2. Steam the diced sweet potatoes until tender.

3. In a bowl, mash the sweet potatoes and mix with black beans, corn, diced tomatoes, chili powder, cumin, salt, and pepper.

4. Place a portion of the mixture in each tortilla, roll them up, and place them seam-side down in a baking dish.

5. Pour the enchilada sauce over the rolled tortillas and sprinkle with vegan shredded cheese.

6. Bake for 20-25 minutes or until the cheese is bubbly and golden.

7. Garnish with fresh cilantro before serving.

Vegan Pad Thai

Ingredients:

- 8 oz (225g) rice noodles
- 1 cup tofu, cubed
- 2 tbsp vegetable oil
- 2 cloves garlic, minced
- 1/2 cup bean sprouts
- 1/4 cup chopped green onions
- 1/4 cup crushed peanuts
- Lime wedges for garnish
- Fresh cilantro for garnish
- Pad Thai sauce (combine 2 tbsp soy sauce, 2 tbsp tamarind paste, 2 tbsp maple syrup, and 1/2 tsp red pepper flakes)

Instructions:

1. Cook rice noodles according to package instructions. Drain and set aside.
2. In a pan, heat vegetable oil and add cubed tofu. Cook until tofu is crispy and golden brown.
3. Add minced garlic and cook for another minute.

4. Add cooked noodles and Pad Thai sauce to the pan. Toss until everything is well combined and heated through.

5. Serve with bean sprouts, chopped green onions, crushed peanuts, lime wedges, and fresh cilantro.

Lentil and Sweet Potato Shepherd's Pie

Ingredients:

- 2 cups cooked green lentils
- 2 cups mashed sweet potatoes
- 1 onion, finely chopped
- 2 cloves garlic, minced
- 1 cup mixed vegetables (carrots, peas, corn)
- 1 cup vegetable broth
- 2 tbsp tomato paste
- 1 tsp thyme
- Salt and pepper to taste
- Olive oil for sautéing

Instructions:

1. Preheat your oven to 375°F (190°C).

2. In a pan, heat olive oil and sauté the onion and garlic until softened.

3. Add mixed vegetables and cook until they start to soften.

4. Stir in cooked green lentils, vegetable broth, tomato paste, thyme, salt, and pepper. Simmer for a few minutes.

5. Transfer the lentil mixture to a baking dish and spread mashed sweet potatoes on top.

6. Bake for 20-25 minutes or until the top is lightly golden.

Vegan Gnocchi with Pesto

Ingredients:

- 1 lb (450g) vegan gnocchi
- 1 cup fresh basil leaves
- 1/2 cup pine nuts
- 2 cloves garlic
- 1/2 cup olive oil
- 1/2 cup nutritional yeast (for a cheesy flavor)

- Salt and pepper to taste

- Cherry tomatoes for garnish (optional)

Instructions:

1. Cook the vegan gnocchi according to package instructions. Drain and set aside.

2. In a food processor, combine fresh basil, pine nuts, garlic, olive oil, nutritional yeast, salt, and pepper. Blend until smooth.

3. Toss the cooked gnocchi with the pesto sauce.

4. Garnish with cherry tomatoes if desired.

Chapter 5: Snacks and Appetizers

When it comes to satisfying those mid-day cravings or impressing guests at a party, having a variety of snacks and appetizers up your sleeve is a must. In this chapter, we'll explore delicious vegan snack and appetizer recipes that are not only easy to prepare but also bursting with flavor.

Guacamole with Veggie Sticks

Ingredients:

- 2 ripe avocados
- 1 small onion, finely diced
- 2 cloves garlic, minced
- 1 tomato, diced
- Juice of 1 lime
- Salt and pepper to taste
- Assorted vegetable sticks (carrots, cucumbers, bell peppers) for dipping

Instructions:

1. Cut the avocados in half, remove the pit, and scoop the flesh into a bowl.

2. Mash the avocados with a fork.

3. Add the diced onion, minced garlic, diced tomato, lime juice, salt, and pepper. Mix until well combined.

4. Serve the guacamole with a platter of assorted vegetable sticks for dipping.

Vegan Spinach and Artichoke Dip

Ingredients:

- 1 cup frozen chopped spinach, thawed and drained
- 1 cup canned artichoke hearts, drained and chopped
- 1 cup vegan cream cheese
- 1/2 cup vegan mayonnaise
- 1/2 cup vegan grated Parmesan cheese
- 1 clove garlic, minced
- Salt and pepper to taste
- Tortilla chips or vegetable sticks for dipping

Instructions:

1. In a mixing bowl, combine the thawed spinach, chopped artichoke hearts, vegan cream cheese, vegan mayonnaise, vegan grated Parmesan cheese, minced garlic, salt, and pepper.
2. Mix until all ingredients are well incorporated.
3. Transfer the mixture to a baking dish and bake at 350°F (175°C) for 25-30 minutes, or until bubbly and slightly golden.
4. Serve with tortilla chips or vegetable sticks.

Hummus with Pita Bread

Ingredients:

- 1 can (15 ounces) chickpeas, drained and rinsed
- 1/4 cup tahini
- 2 cloves garlic, minced
- Juice of 1 lemon
- 2 tablespoons olive oil
- 1/2 teaspoon cumin
- Salt and pepper to taste
- Pita bread, cut into triangles for dipping

Instructions:

1. In a food processor, combine the chickpeas, tahini, minced garlic, lemon juice, olive oil, cumin, salt, and pepper.
2. Blend until smooth and creamy, adding a bit of water if needed to reach the desired consistency.
3. Serve the hummus with pita bread triangles for dipping.

Vegan Salsa Verde

Ingredients:

- 6 tomatillos, husked and rinsed
- 1 jalapeño pepper, seeds removed (adjust to taste)
- 1/2 onion, chopped
- 2 cloves garlic
- 1/2 cup fresh cilantro leaves
- Juice of 1 lime
- Salt to taste
- Tortilla chips for serving

Instructions:

1. In a blender, combine the tomatillos, jalapeño pepper, chopped onion, garlic, cilantro, lime juice, and salt.
2. Blend until you achieve a smooth salsa verde.
3. Refrigerate for at least 30 minutes before serving with tortilla chips.

Sweet Potato Fries

Ingredients:

- 2 large sweet potatoes, peeled and cut into fries
- 2 tablespoons olive oil
- 1 teaspoon paprika
- 1/2 teaspoon garlic powder
- Salt and pepper to taste

Instructions:

1. Preheat your oven to 425°F (220°C).
2. In a large bowl, toss the sweet potato fries with olive oil, paprika, garlic powder, salt, and pepper until they are evenly coated.

3. Spread the fries out on a baking sheet in a single layer.

4. Bake for 20-25 minutes or until the fries are crispy and golden brown, flipping them halfway through.

Vegan Buffalo Cauliflower Bites

Ingredients:

- 1 head of cauliflower, cut into florets
- 1 cup almond milk
- 1 cup all-purpose flour
- 1 teaspoon garlic powder
- 1 teaspoon paprika
- 1/2 cup vegan buffalo sauce
- Vegan ranch or blue cheese dressing for dipping

Instructions:

1. Preheat your oven to 450°F (230°C).

2. In a mixing bowl, whisk together almond milk, all-purpose flour, garlic powder, and paprika until you have a smooth batter.

3. Dip each cauliflower floret into the batter, ensuring it's fully coated, and then place it on a baking sheet.

4. Bake for 20-25 minutes or until the cauliflower is crispy and slightly browned.

5. Toss the baked cauliflower in vegan buffalo sauce.

6. Serve with vegan ranch or blue cheese dressing for dipping.

Stuffed Mushrooms

Ingredients:

- 18 large white mushrooms, stems removed and reserved
- 1/2 cup vegan cream cheese
- 1/4 cup breadcrumbs
- 2 cloves garlic, minced
- 2 tablespoons fresh parsley, chopped
- Salt and pepper to taste
- Olive oil for drizzling

Instructions:

1. Preheat your oven to 375°F (190°C).

2. Chop the mushroom stems finely.

3. In a mixing bowl, combine the chopped mushroom stems, vegan cream cheese, breadcrumbs, minced garlic, chopped parsley, salt, and pepper.

4. Stuff each mushroom cap with this mixture.

5. Place the stuffed mushrooms on a baking sheet, drizzle with olive oil, and bake for 20-25 minutes until the mushrooms are tender and the stuffing is golden.

Vegan Spring Rolls

Ingredients:
- Rice paper wrappers
- 2 cups cooked rice noodles
- Assorted veggies (carrots, cucumber, bell peppers, lettuce)
- Fresh herbs (mint, basil)
- Vegan hoisin or peanut dipping sauce

Instructions:
1. Prepare a shallow dish of warm water.

2. Dip a rice paper wrapper into the warm water for a few seconds until it softens.

3. Lay the softened wrapper flat on a clean surface.

4. Place a handful of cooked rice noodles and a mix of your favorite veggies and herbs on the lower half of the wrapper.

5. Fold the sides of the wrapper in and roll it up tightly.

6. Repeat with the remaining wrappers and filling.

7. Serve with vegan hoisin or peanut dipping sauce.

Roasted Chickpeas

Ingredients:

- 2 cans (15 ounces each) chickpeas, drained and rinsed
- 2 tablespoons olive oil
- 1 teaspoon smoked paprika
- 1/2 teaspoon cumin
- Salt and pepper to taste

Instructions:

1. Preheat your oven to 400°F (200°C).

2. Pat the chickpeas dry with a paper towel.

3. In a bowl, toss the chickpeas with olive oil, smoked paprika, cumin, salt, and pepper until well coated.

4. Spread them out on a baking sheet and roast for 25-
    30 minutes or until crispy, shaking the pan
    occasionally.

Vegan Caprese Skewers

Ingredients:

- Cherry tomatoes
- Vegan mozzarella-style cheese, cut into small cubes
- Fresh basil leaves
- Balsamic glaze for drizzling
- Skewers or toothpicks

Instructions:

1. Thread a cherry tomato, a cube of vegan mozzarella,
    and a fresh basil leaf onto each skewer or toothpick.
2. Arrange the skewers on a platter.
3. Drizzle with balsamic glaze just before serving.

Vegan Popcorn with Nutritional Yeast

Ingredients:

- Popcorn kernels
- 2 tablespoons nutritional yeast
- 1 tablespoon olive oil
- Salt to taste

Instructions:

1. Pop the popcorn kernels using your preferred method (stove, microwave, or air popper).
2. Drizzle olive oil over the popped popcorn and toss to coat.
3. Sprinkle nutritional yeast and salt over the popcorn, and toss again until well seasoned.

Spicy Vegan Nuts

Ingredients:

- 2 cups mixed nuts (almonds, cashews, peanuts, etc.)
- 2 tablespoons olive oil
- 1 teaspoon paprika

- 1/2 teaspoon cayenne pepper (adjust to taste)
- 1/2 teaspoon garlic powder
- Salt to taste

Instructions:

1. Preheat your oven to 350°F (175°C).
2. In a bowl, toss the mixed nuts with olive oil, paprika, cayenne pepper, garlic powder, and salt until evenly coated.
3. Spread the seasoned nuts on a baking sheet and roast for 10-15 minutes, or until they become fragrant and slightly crispy. Keep an eye on them to prevent burning.

Vegan Bruschetta

Ingredients:

- Baguette or Italian bread, sliced
- 4-5 ripe tomatoes, diced
- 1/4 cup fresh basil leaves, chopped
- 2 cloves garlic, minced
- 2 tablespoons balsamic vinegar
- 2 tablespoons olive oil

- Salt and pepper to taste

Instructions:

1. Toast the bread slices in the oven or on a grill until they are lightly browned.

2. In a bowl, combine the diced tomatoes, chopped basil, minced garlic, balsamic vinegar, olive oil, salt, and pepper.

3. Spoon the tomato mixture onto the toasted bread slices.

Vegan Cucumber Rolls

Ingredients:

- Cucumbers
- Vegan cream cheese
- Sliced bell peppers, carrots, and avocado
- Fresh herbs (parsley, cilantro)
- Salt and pepper to taste

Instructions:

1. Slice the cucumbers lengthwise into thin strips using a mandoline or a vegetable peeler.

2. Spread vegan cream cheese on each cucumber strip.

3. Place a slice of bell pepper, carrot, and avocado on each strip.

4. Add a sprig of fresh herbs.

5. Sprinkle with salt and pepper to taste.

6. Roll up the cucumber strips and secure with a toothpick.

Vegan Onion Rings

Ingredients:

- 2 large onions, cut into rings
- 1 cup all-purpose flour
- 1 cup almond milk
- 1 teaspoon paprika
- 1 teaspoon garlic powder
- Salt and pepper to taste
- Vegetable oil for frying

Instructions:

1. In a bowl, whisk together the flour, almond milk, paprika, garlic powder, salt, and pepper to create a batter.

2. Dip the onion rings into the batter to coat them.

3. Heat vegetable oil in a deep frying pan or a deep fryer.

4. Fry the coated onion rings until they are golden brown and crispy.

5. Remove and drain on paper towels.

Vegan Nachos

Ingredients:

- Tortilla chips
- Vegan cheese sauce or shredded vegan cheese
- Black beans, drained and rinsed
- Sliced black olives
- Sliced jalapeños
- Diced tomatoes
- Vegan sour cream and guacamole for dipping

Instructions:

1. Arrange the tortilla chips on a serving platter.

2. Drizzle with vegan cheese sauce or sprinkle with shredded vegan cheese.

3. Top with black beans, black olives, jalapeños, and diced tomatoes.

4. Serve with vegan sour cream and guacamole for dipping.

Vegan Potato Skins

Ingredients:

- 4 large russet potatoes
- 2 tablespoons olive oil
- 1 cup vegan cheddar cheese, shredded
- Vegan sour cream
- Chopped green onions
- Salt and pepper to taste

Instructions:

1. Scrub and bake the potatoes until they are tender. Let them cool slightly.

2. Cut each potato in half lengthwise and scoop out the flesh, leaving about 1/4 inch of potato on the skin.

3. Brush the potato skins with olive oil and season with salt and pepper.

4. Place the skins on a baking sheet and bake until crispy.

5. Remove from the oven and sprinkle with vegan cheddar cheese.

6. Return to the oven until the cheese is melted and bubbly.

7. Serve with vegan sour cream and chopped green onions.

Vegan Tofu Satay

Ingredients:

- Extra-firm tofu, cubed
- 1/4 cup soy sauce
- 2 tablespoons peanut butter
- 2 tablespoons lime juice
- 1 tablespoon maple syrup
- 1 clove garlic, minced
- Skewers or toothpicks

Instructions:

1. In a bowl, whisk together soy sauce, peanut butter, lime juice, maple syrup, and minced garlic to make the marinade.
2. Thread the cubed tofu onto skewers or toothpicks.
3. Brush the tofu with the marinade and let it sit for at least 30 minutes.
4. Grill or pan-fry the tofu skewers until they are browned and slightly crispy.
5. Serve with extra marinade for dipping.

Chapter 6: Desserts

Indulging in a sweet treat doesn't have to mean sacrificing your commitment to a vegan lifestyle. In this chapter, we've gathered an array of delectable vegan desserts that will satisfy your cravings and delight your taste buds. From rich and creamy to fruity and light, these recipes ensure you can enjoy dessert while staying true to your values.

Vegan Chocolate Avocado Mousse

Ingredients:

- 2 ripe avocados
- 1/4 cup cocoa powder
- 1/4 cup maple syrup
- 1 tsp vanilla extract
- A pinch of salt

Instructions:

1. Scoop the flesh of the avocados into a blender.
2. Add cocoa powder, maple syrup, vanilla extract, and a pinch of salt.

3. Blend until smooth and creamy.

4. Refrigerate for an hour before serving. Garnish with berries if desired.

Vegan Banana Bread

Ingredients:

- 3 ripe bananas
- 1/4 cup coconut oil
- 1/2 cup maple syrup
- 1 tsp vanilla extract
- 1 1/2 cups whole wheat flour
- 1 tsp baking soda
- A pinch of salt
- 1/2 cup chopped walnuts (optional)

Instructions:

1. Preheat your oven to 350°F (175°C). Grease a loaf pan.

2. Mash the ripe bananas in a bowl.

3. Stir in coconut oil, maple syrup, and vanilla extract.

4. In a separate bowl, mix whole wheat flour, baking soda, and a pinch of salt.

5. Combine the wet and dry ingredients. Fold in chopped walnuts.

6. Pour the batter into the loaf pan and bake for about 45 minutes.

7. Allow to cool before slicing.

Berry Crisp

Ingredients:

- 4 cups mixed berries (strawberries, blueberries, raspberries)
- 1 cup rolled oats
- 1/2 cup almond meal
- 1/4 cup maple syrup
- 1/4 cup coconut oil
- 1 tsp cinnamon
- A pinch of salt

Instructions:

1. Preheat your oven to 350°F (175°C).

2. In a bowl, combine mixed berries with 2 tbsp of maple syrup. Pour into a baking dish.

3. In another bowl, mix rolled oats, almond meal, remaining maple syrup, melted coconut oil, cinnamon, and a pinch of salt.

4. Sprinkle the oat mixture evenly over the berries.

5. Bake for 30-35 minutes or until the topping is golden brown and the berries are bubbling.

6. Serve warm.

Vegan Chocolate Chip Cookies

Ingredients:

- 1 1/2 cups all-purpose flour
- 1/2 tsp baking soda
- 1/2 cup vegan butter
- 1/2 cup brown sugar
- 1/4 cup white sugar
- 1 tsp vanilla extract
- 1/4 cup unsweetened applesauce
- 1 cup vegan chocolate chips

Instructions:

1. Preheat your oven to 350°F (175°C). Grease a baking sheet.

2. In a bowl, whisk together flour and baking soda.

3. In another bowl, cream vegan butter, brown sugar, and white sugar until well combined.

4. Stir in vanilla extract and applesauce.

5. Gradually add the dry ingredients to the wet mixture and mix until a dough forms.

6. Fold in the vegan chocolate chips.

7. Drop spoonfuls of dough onto the baking sheet and bake for 10-12 minutes until edges are golden.

Vegan Rice Pudding

Ingredients:

- 1 cup Arborio rice
- 4 cups almond milk
- 1/3 cup maple syrup
- 1 tsp vanilla extract
- 1/2 tsp ground cinnamon
- A pinch of salt

Instructions:

1. Rinse the Arborio rice and drain.

2. In a saucepan, combine rice, almond milk, maple syrup, vanilla extract, ground cinnamon, and a pinch of salt.

3. Bring to a simmer over low heat and cook, stirring occasionally, for 30-40 minutes until the rice is tender and the mixture thickens.

4. Remove from heat, let it cool slightly, and serve warm or chilled.

Vegan Blueberry Cheesecake

Ingredients:

- 1 1/2 cups cashews (soaked)
- 1/2 cup coconut cream
- 1/4 cup lemon juice
- 1/4 cup maple syrup
- 1 tsp vanilla extract
- 1 cup fresh or frozen blueberries
- 1 1/2 cups almond meal and dates for the crust

Instructions:

1. Blend soaked cashews, coconut cream, lemon juice, maple syrup, and vanilla extract until smooth.

2. In a separate bowl, combine almond meal and dates. Press this mixture into the base of a cheesecake pan.

3. Pour the cashew mixture over the crust.

4. Swirl in the blueberries.

5. Freeze for 4-6 hours until set.

Vegan Apple Crumble

Ingredients:

- 4 cups sliced apples
- 1 tbsp lemon juice
- 1/2 cup rolled oats
- 1/2 cup almond meal
- 1/4 cup maple syrup
- 2 tbsp coconut oil
- 1 tsp cinnamon
- A pinch of salt

Instructions:

1. Preheat your oven to 350°F (175°C). Grease a baking dish.

2. Toss sliced apples with lemon juice and place them in the baking dish.

3. In a bowl, combine rolled oats, almond meal, maple syrup, melted coconut oil, cinnamon, and a pinch of salt.

4. Sprinkle the oat mixture evenly over the apples.

5. Bake for 30-35 minutes or until the topping is golden and the apples are tender.

Chocolate Covered Strawberries

Ingredients:
- Fresh strawberries
- Vegan chocolate chips
- Coconut oil (optional)

Instructions:
1. Wash and dry the strawberries thoroughly.

2. In a microwave-safe bowl, melt vegan chocolate chips in 20-second intervals, stirring between each, until smooth. Add a small amount of coconut oil if desired for smoother consistency.

3. Dip each strawberry into the melted chocolate, letting excess drip off.

4. Place the chocolate-covered strawberries on a parchment-lined tray.

5. Refrigerate until the chocolate hardens.

Vegan Pumpkin Pie

Ingredients:

- 1 1/2 cups pumpkin puree
- 1/2 cup coconut milk
- 1/2 cup maple syrup
- 1 tsp cinnamon
- 1/2 tsp nutmeg
- 1/4 tsp ginger
- 1/4 tsp cloves
- A pinch of salt
- Vegan pie crust

Instructions:

1. Preheat your oven to 350°F (175°C).

2. In a bowl, mix pumpkin puree, coconut milk, maple syrup, spices, and a pinch of salt until well combined.

3. Pour the mixture into a prepared vegan pie crust.

4. Bake for 45-50 minutes or until the pie is set.

5. Let it cool before serving.

Vegan Coconut Macaroons

Ingredients:

- 2 1/2 cups shredded coconut
- 1/2 cup almond flour
- 1/2 cup maple syrup
- 1/4 cup coconut oil
- 1 tsp vanilla extract
- A pinch of salt
- Vegan chocolate for drizzling (optional)

Instructions:

1. Preheat your oven to 350°F (175°C). Line a baking sheet with parchment paper.
2. In a bowl, combine shredded coconut, almond flour, maple syrup, melted coconut oil, vanilla extract, and a pinch of salt.
3. Scoop spoonfuls of the mixture onto the baking sheet.
4. Bake for 12-15 minutes or until golden brown.

5. Let the macaroons cool. Optionally, drizzle with melted vegan chocolate.

Vegan Chocolate Fondue

Ingredients:

- 1 cup vegan chocolate chips
- 1/2 cup coconut milk
- Assorted fruits (strawberries, bananas, pineapple) and marshmallows for dipping

Instructions:

1. In a saucepan, heat coconut milk until it starts to simmer.
2. Remove from heat and stir in vegan chocolate chips until smooth.
3. Transfer the mixture to a fondue pot or a serving bowl.
4. Dip your favorite fruits and marshmallows into the warm chocolate fondue.

Vegan Lemon Bars

Ingredients:

- 1 1/2 cups almond flour
- 1/4 cup maple syrup
- 1/4 cup coconut oil
- 1 cup lemon juice
- Zest of one lemon
- 1/2 cup coconut cream
- 1/4 cup arrowroot powder
- Powdered sugar for dusting (optional)

Instructions:

1. Preheat your oven to 350°F (175°C). Grease a baking dish.
2. In a bowl, combine almond flour, maple syrup, and melted coconut oil.
3. Press this mixture into the base of the baking dish and bake for 12-15 minutes until lightly golden.
4. In another bowl, whisk together lemon juice, lemon zest, coconut cream, and arrowroot powder until smooth.
5. Pour the lemon mixture over the baked crust.

6. Bake for another 20-25 minutes until set.

7. Let it cool and optionally dust with powdered sugar.

Vegan Peanut Butter Cups

Ingredients:

- 1/2 cup vegan chocolate chips

- 1/4 cup peanut butter

- 2 tbsp maple syrup

Instructions:

1. In a microwave-safe bowl, melt half of the vegan chocolate chips in 20-second intervals, stirring between each, until smooth.

2. Spoon a small amount of melted chocolate into mini muffin cup liners and spread it to coat the bottom and sides.

3. Place in the freezer to set.

4. In another bowl, mix peanut butter and maple syrup.

5. Spoon the peanut butter mixture into the chocolate cups.

6. Melt the remaining chocolate chips and spoon it over the peanut butter to cover.

7. Freeze until set.

Vegan Strawberry Shortcake

Ingredients:

- 1 cup fresh strawberries, sliced
- 1 cup all-purpose flour
- 1/4 cup sugar
- 1 tsp baking powder
- 1/2 tsp baking soda
- 1/4 cup coconut oil
- 1/2 cup almond milk
- 1 tsp vanilla extract
- Vegan whipped cream (optional)

Instructions:

1. Preheat your oven to 350°F (175°C). Grease a cake pan.
2. In a bowl, mix flour, sugar, baking powder, and baking soda.
3. In a separate bowl, combine melted coconut oil, almond milk, and vanilla extract.

4. Add the wet mixture to the dry ingredients and stir until combined.

5. Pour the batter into the cake pan and bake for 20-25 minutes or until a toothpick comes out clean.

6. Let the cake cool, then slice it in half horizontally.

7. Layer the bottom half with sliced strawberries and vegan whipped cream if desired. Top with the other cake half and more strawberries.

Vegan Carrot Cake

Ingredients:

- 2 cups grated carrots
- 1 1/2 cups all-purpose flour
- 1 tsp baking powder
- 1/2 tsp baking soda
- 1/2 tsp cinnamon
- 1/4 tsp nutmeg
- 1/4 cup coconut oil
- 1/2 cup maple syrup
- 1/4 cup applesauce
- 1 tsp vanilla extract
- 1/2 cup crushed pineapple, drained

- 1/2 cup chopped walnuts (optional)
- Vegan cream cheese frosting (store-bought or homemade)

Instructions:

1. Preheat your oven to 350°F (175°C). Grease a cake pan.
2. In a bowl, whisk together flour, baking powder, baking soda, cinnamon, and nutmeg.
3. In another bowl, mix melted coconut oil, maple syrup, applesauce, and vanilla extract.
4. Add the wet mixture to the dry ingredients and stir until combined.
5. Fold in grated carrots, crushed pineapple, and chopped walnuts (if using).
6. Pour the batter into the cake pan and bake for 25-30 minutes or until a toothpick comes out clean.
7. Let the cake cool and frost with vegan cream cheese frosting.

Vegan Chocolate Pots de Crème

Ingredients:

- 1 cup full-fat coconut milk
- 1/4 cup cocoa powder
- 1/4 cup maple syrup
- 1/2 cup vegan chocolate chips
- 1 tsp vanilla extract
- A pinch of salt

Instructions:

1. In a saucepan, heat coconut milk, cocoa powder, maple syrup, and a pinch of salt until it starts to simmer.
2. Remove from heat and stir in vegan chocolate chips and vanilla extract until smooth.
3. Pour the mixture into serving glasses.
4. Refrigerate for a few hours or until set.

Vegan Black Bean Brownies

Ingredients:

- 1 can (15 oz) black beans, drained and rinsed

- 1/4 cup cocoa powder
- 1/2 cup maple syrup
- 1/4 cup coconut oil
- 1 tsp vanilla extract
- 1/2 cup vegan chocolate chips

Instructions:

1. Preheat your oven to 350°F (175°C). Grease a baking dish.
2. In a blender, combine black beans, cocoa powder, maple syrup, melted coconut oil, and vanilla extract until smooth.
3. Stir in vegan chocolate chips.
4. Pour the batter into the baking dish and bake for 15-20 minutes or until a toothpick comes out with a few moist crumbs.
5. Let it cool before cutting into squares.

Vegan Tiramisu

(Note: Tiramisu typically contains coffee and mascarpone, which are not vegan. This vegan version uses alternatives.)

Ingredients:

- 1 cup strong brewed coffee (cooled)
- 1 package vegan ladyfingers
- 1 cup vegan cream cheese
- 1/2 cup coconut cream
- 1/4 cup powdered sugar
- 1 tsp vanilla extract
- Cocoa powder for dusting

Instructions:

1. Dip ladyfingers into brewed coffee and arrange them in a serving dish.
2. In a bowl, whisk together vegan cream cheese, coconut cream, powdered sugar, and vanilla extract until smooth.
3. Spread a layer of the cream mixture over the ladyfingers.

4. Repeat the layers, finishing with a layer of cream on
   top.

5. Refrigerate for a few hours or overnight.

6. Dust with cocoa powder before serving.

CONCLUSION

As we embark on the final chapter of this culinary journey towards better renal health, it's essential to reflect on the path we've walked together. The recipes and meal plans shared in this book aren't just about food; they represent a commitment to your well-being, a dedication to nurturing your body, and a celebration of the vibrant flavors that a vegan diet can offer.

Throughout this book, we've explored the intricate balance of flavors, textures, and nutrients that can be achieved through plant-based cooking. We've delved into creative breakfasts, hearty lunches, satisfying dinners, tantalizing snacks, and indulgent desserts, all while keeping your renal health at the forefront

But this isn't just the end; it's a new beginning. Your journey toward improved renal health is ongoing, and these recipes are just a stepping stone. Remember, a plant-based diet isn't a one-size-fits-all solution, and it's crucial to consult with a healthcare professional to tailor your dietary choices to your specific needs.

In this concluding chapter, we invite you to take the knowledge and inspiration you've gained from this book and apply it to your daily life. Experiment with these recipes, adapt them to your preferences, and explore new flavors and ingredients. Discover the joy of cooking and sharing these meals with loved ones. Most importantly, prioritize your health and well-being.

As you move forward, remember that every meal is an opportunity to nourish your body and support your renal health. It's a chance to savor the deliciousness of plant-based cuisine while making a positive impact on your overall well-being. Your journey toward renal health is a testament to your dedication to a healthier you, and this book is here to support you every step of the way.

Thank you for embarking on this flavorful adventure with us. Here's to your health, happiness, and the vibrant world of vegan cooking that awaits you beyond these pages.

www.ingramcontent.com/pod-product-compliance
Lightning Source LLC
Chambersburg PA
CBHW070811260726
48660CB00005B/1803